Mental Health Nursing
Practical Record Book
for
BSc Nursing and PB BSc Nursing

Mental Health Nursing
Practical Record Book
for
BSc Nursing and PB BSc Nursing

As per the INC Syllabus

Third Edition

R Sreevani PhD (Psychiatric Nursing)
Professor and Head
Department of Psychiatric Nursing
Dharwad Institute of Mental Health and Neurosciences (DIMHANS)
Dharwad, Karnataka, India

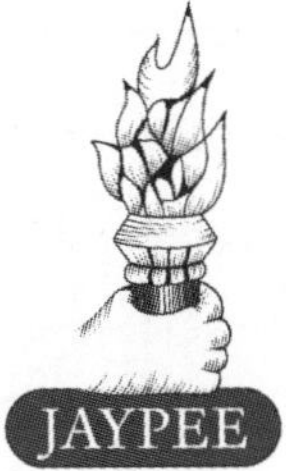

JAYPEE

JAYPEE BROTHERS MEDICAL PUBLISHERS
The Health Sciences Publisher
New Delhi | London

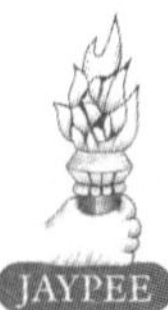 **Jaypee Brothers Medical Publishers (P) Ltd.**

Headquarters

Jaypee Brothers Medical Publishers (P) Ltd.
EMCA House, 23/23-B
Ansari Road, Daryaganj
New Delhi 110 002, India
Landline: +91-11-23272143, +91-11-23272703
+91-11-23282021, +91-11-23245672
Email: jaypee@jaypeebrothers.com

Corporate Office

Jaypee Brothers Medical Publishers (P) Ltd.
4838/24, Ansari Road, Daryaganj
New Delhi 110 002, India
Phone: +91-11-43574357
Fax: +91-11-43574314
Email: jaypee@jaypeebrothers.com

Website: www.jaypeebrothers.com
Website: www.jaypeedigital.com

EU GPSR Authorised Representative
Logos Europe, 9 rue Nicolas Poussin
17000, La Rochelle, France
Phone: +33 (0) 6 67 93 73 78
E-mail: Contact@logoseurope.eu

Overseas Office
JP Medical Ltd.
83, Victoria Street, London
SW1H 0HW (UK)
Phone: +44-20 3170 8910
Fax: +44(0)20 3008 6180
E-mail: info@jpmedpub.com

Inquiries for bulk sales may be solicited at: jaypee@jaypeebrothers.com

Mental Health Nursing Practical Record Book for BSc Nursing and PB BSc Nursing

First Edition: 2011

Second Edition: 2017

Third Edition: **2024**

Reprint: **2025**

ISBN: 978-93-5696-650-5

Printed in India at Purewall Ventures Pvt Ltd

Preface

Mental health nurses work with people suffering from various mental health conditions and also their caregivers. Their work involves helping the patients in not only recovering from their illness but also coming to terms with the illness in order to lead a positive life. They often work in multidisciplinary teams, liaising with psychiatrists, psychologists, occupational therapists, social workers, and other health professionals.

As a mental health nurse, he/she is required to deal with acute and chronic patients in a variety of settings which may range from community healthcare centers to hospital outpatient and inpatient departments. In order to play her varied role in an effective manner, it is imperative that the mental health nurse is both knowledgeable and competent. Toward achieving this end, the nurse is required to gain expertise in both theoretical and clinical areas.

During my teaching experience at both undergraduate and graduate levels, I observed that the students are submitting their assignments in loose sheets and later collating them, thus giving a muddled appearance. Moreover, the nursing students do not have any standard formats to look to, resulting in compiling the information in a haphazard manner and also omitting the basic information in certain instances. This *Practical Record Book* has been designed with a basic idea to redress such issues.

There has been a genuine effort on my part to design the record in such a way as to help the student document the necessary information in a systematic and scientific manner. It not only includes the outline of various assignments to be completed by the students during their psychiatric clinical experience postings but also fulfils the clinical experience as prescribed by the revised Indian Nursing Council (INC) syllabus. Notes on a few topics have also been provided at the beginning to assist the student-nurses.

I sincerely hope that this publication will help the student-nurses achieve essential skills and also the desired results in their examinations.

R Sreevani

Clinical Experience Record of Mental Health Nursing

Name of the student :...

Register No. :...

Year :...

Name and address of the institution :...

....

....

....

....

Name of the hospital/nursing home (where the mental health nursing clinical practice attended) :...

....

....

....

....

....

Photograph

Signature of Student

Date:

Signature of Class Coordinator

Date:

Signature of HOD

Date:

Signature of Principal

Date:

Clinical Requirements for V and VI Semester BSc Nursing as per Indian Nursing Council

S. No.	Areas	Assignment number	Nursing procedure	Recommended	Completed
1.	Psychiatric OPD	1	Objectives, philosophy and physical set-up of the mental hospital/nursing home/institution	1	
		2 and 3	History taking and mental status examination	2	
		4	Assisting psychometric assessment	1	
		5	Neurological examination	1	
		6	Health education	1	
		7	Observational report of OPD	1	
2.	Child guidance clinic	8	Care plan (child psychiatric ward)	1	
		9	Observational report of different therapies	1	
3.	Inpatient ward	10	Case study	1	
		11, 12,13	Care plan	3	
		14	Clinical presentation	1	
		15 and 16	Process recording	2	
		17, 18, 19	Administration of medications for 3 patients	3	
		20	Assist electroconvulsive therapy (ECT)	1	
			Assist/participate in all therapies		
		21	◆ Individual psychotherapy	1	
		22	◆ Family psychotherapy	1	
		23	◆ Group psychotherapy	1	
		24	◆ Occupational therapy	1	
		25	◆ Behavioral therapy	1	
		26	◆ Recreational therapy	1	
		27	◆ Play therapy	1	
		28, 29, 30	Prepare the patients for activities of daily living for 3 patients	3	
		31	Admission procedure	1	
		32	Discharge procedure	1	
		33	Health education	1	
		34	Drug book (minimum 20 drugs)		
4.	Community psychiatry	35	Community case work	1	
		36	Observational report on field visits		
		37	Observational report on de-addiction center	1	

This is to certify that he /she has completed clinical requirements as per the prescribed syllabus.

Signature of Student   Signature of Class Coordinator   Signature of Subject Teacher   Signature of HOD

Date: Date: Date: Date:

Signature of Internal Examiner   Signature of External Examiner

Date: Date:

Contents

Short Notes on Nursing Process in Psychiatric Nursing

DEFINITION

Nursing process is an orderly, systematic manner of determining the patient's problems, making plans to solve them, initiating the plan or assigning others to implement it and evaluating the extent to which the plan was effective in resolving the problems identified.

—Yura and Walsh, 1978

Steps in the nursing process supply an organized approach for providing quality psychiatric mental health nursing care. The five steps involved are the same as those used in other nursing specialties such as medical-surgical nursing, maternity nursing and pediatric nursing. Differences for this specialty however exist in terms of the manner and focus of the nurse's observations, particulars of interviewing during data collection and the types of interventions used for identifying problems.

The five steps in nursing process are **(Fig. 1)**:
1. Assessment or gathering data
2. Diagnosis or identifying a problem
3. Planning or creating a plan to achieve desired outcomes
4. Implementation or enacting the plan
5. Evaluation or determining the effectiveness of the plan

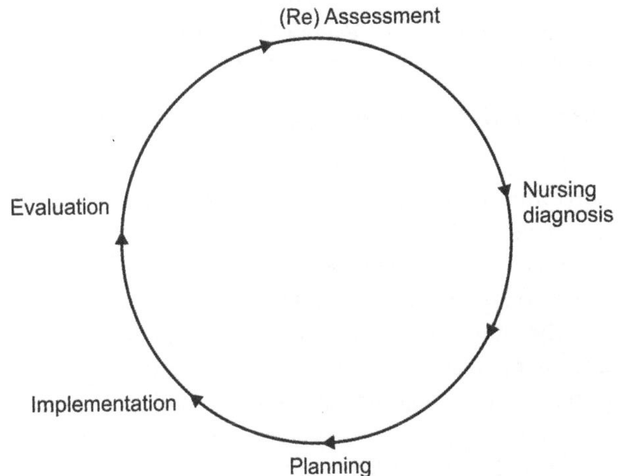

Fig. 1: Steps in nursing process

NURSING ASSESSMENT

Assessment involves the collection, organization and analysis of information about the patient's health. In psychiatric mental health nursing, this process is often referred to as psychosocial assessment. The nurse obtains assessment data from several sources **(Box 1)**.

Box 1: Components of psychosocial assessment	
◆ Interview with the patient and his family ◆ History and physical examination ◆ Mental status examination	◆ Records from other health care facilities or prior treatment ◆ Laboratory and psychological tests ◆ Assessment by other professionals and paraprofessionals

CLINICAL INTERVIEW

Interview allows the nurse to hear patient's perspective on the problem **(Box 2)**.

Box 2: Effective interview skills	
◆ Conduct the interview in a quiet place, ensure privacy ◆ Be relaxed and maintain an unhurried posture ◆ Maintain eye contact with the patient ◆ Be interested and attentive to what he says ◆ Pick-up verbal and nonverbal cues of distress ◆ Allow the patient to talk freely without any interruption	◆ When the patient deviates from the theme or loses his track, guide him to the main theme politely ◆ Use open-ended questions ◆ Use active listening ◆ Do not offer premature conclusions and assurance on the outcome of the treatment

▌HISTORY TAKING

History taking and mental status examination are core clinical skills of psychiatry. History taking should be collected under the following categories:

Identification and Demographical Details

This includes patient's name, age, sex, religion, address, socioeconomic status, hospital number, marital status, occupation, details of informant, and information relevant or not, adequate or not.

Presenting Complaints/Chief Complaints

Here symptoms are listed in a chronological order with their duration. Sometimes the patient may deny the existence of any symptoms and say that he was forcibly brought to the hospital by his relatives. In such cases, information is collected from his relatives. It is preferable to use patient's own words verbatim, without translating or interpreting their meaning. For example, sleeplessness—3 weeks, loss of appetite and hearing voices—2 weeks.

History of Present Illness

Under this are recorded the evolution of patient's symptoms from the time they were first noted till the time of consultation. Details of each symptom should be collected. Patient's history may have to be supplemented with data available from other sources.

It is ideal to use patient's own words. Look for and also ask for any precipitating factors. An attempt should also be made to identify any possible secondary gain to the patient because of his symptoms.

The mode of onset of illness may be acute or insidious. Progress may be steady and progressive or diminishing and reappearing periodically or staying the same way throughout. These should also be enquired into. Sometimes the patient is able to point out some antecedent stressful event alluded as precipitants. Temporal relation of the event with illness, severity of the stress, patient's preoccupation with the events and the value attached to the event by him may all give a clue to the presence and nature of the precipitant.

Past Psychiatric History

Enquire whether the patient had any psychiatric illness in the past. If so its nature, duration, treatment and outcome should be noted down. If treatment was discontinued in the middle enquire the reason for this as well as the reason for switching over to other models of therapy.

Family History

Enquire about the type and size of family and the general family environment. The presence of psychiatric illness on the paternal or maternal side should be routinely asked. It would be useful to construct a family tree depicting the living members, their age, deceased members and their age at death. Mark whether any of them has or had similar illness and if known, the type of treatment they received and the outcome. Note specifically any history of suicide, mental retardation, epilepsy or any genetically transmittable disorders **(Fig. 2)**.

Personal History

Personal history includes the developmental, educational, occupational as well as the sexual history of the patient. Developmental history includes details of pregnancy and delivery, developmental milestones, health during childhood and adolescence, neurotic symptoms and occurrence of any significant event (e.g., separation from parents, bereavements, etc., are recorded). Educational history relates to details regarding the level of performance in school, relationship with peers and teachers, academic achievements and extracurricular activities. While collecting occupational history, enquiry should be made about the types of work, job satisfaction, whether jobs were changed frequently and if so, reasons thereof, work skills and relationship with colleagues. Sexual history includes details about sexual development, practices and attitudes towards sex. In marital history enquiry should be made about married life and details about spouse and children.

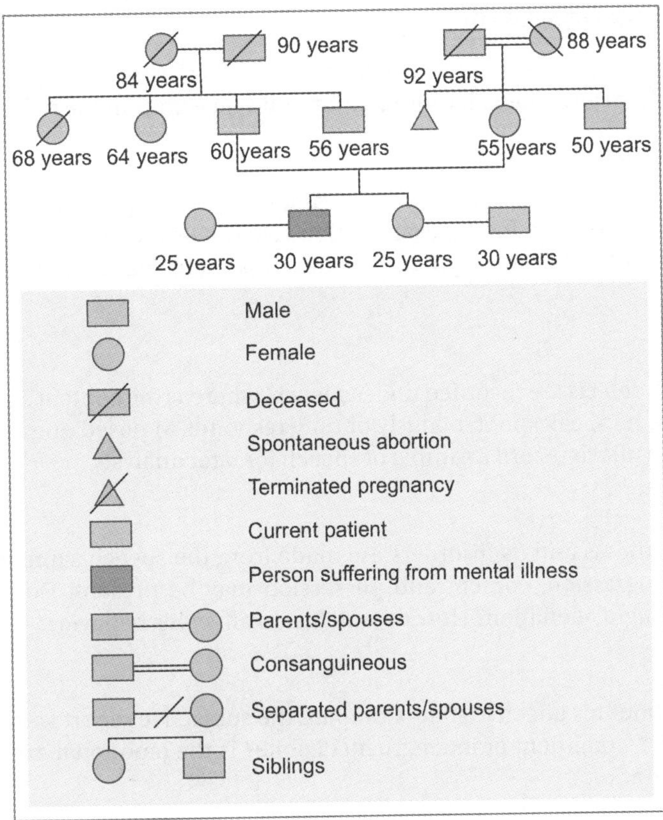

Fig. 2: Family genogram

Premorbid Personality

Personality of a patient consists of those habitual attitudes and patterns of behavior which characterize an individual. Personality sometimes changes after the onset of illness. The nurse has to get a description of the personality before the onset of illness and aim to build up a picture of the individual, not a type. Enquiry in the following areas has to be made:

- **Attitude to others in social, family and sexual relationship:** Ability to trust others, make and sustain relationships, anxious or secure, leader or follower, level of participation, ability to take up responsibility, capacity to make a decision, dominant or submissive, friendly or emotionally cold, etc. Difficulty in role taking—gender, sexual and familial.
- **Attitude to self:** Egocentric, selfish, indulgent, dramatizing, critical, depreciatory, over concerned, self-conscious, satisfaction or dissatisfaction with work. Attitude towards health and bodily functions. Attitude to past achievements and failure, and to the future.
- **Moral and religious attitudes and standards:** Evidence of rigidity or compliance, permissiveness or over conscientiousness, conformity or rebellion. Enquire specifically about religious beliefs. Excessive religiosity.
- **Mood:** Enquire about stability of mood, mood swings, whether anxious, irritable, worrying or tense. Whether lively or gloomy. Ability to express and control feelings of anger, anxiety or depression.
- **Leisure activities and hobbies:** Interest in reading, playing, music, movies, etc. Enquire about creative ability. Whether leisure time is spent alone or with friends. Is the circle of friends large or small?
- **Fantasy life:** Enquire about content of day dreams and dreams. Amount of time spent in day dreaming.
- **Reaction pattern to stress:** Ability to tolerate frustrations, losses, disappointments and circumstances arousing anger, anxiety or depression. Evidence for the excessive use of particular defense mechanisms such as denial, rationalization, projection, etc.

MENTAL STATUS EXAMINATION (MSE)

Mental status examination is used to determine whether a patient is experiencing abnormalities in thinking and reasoning ability, feelings or behavior. It includes observations and questions in the following categories:

General Appearance and Behavior

Describe patient's appearance and behavior. Is he dressed properly? Assess patient's sensorium. Is he alert? Drowsy? Stuporous? Comatose? Is he co-operative for the examination? Does he make eye contact with the examiner? What is his level of activity? Is he excited? Retarded? Hyperactive? Restless? Does he have any mannerisms? Gestures? Tics? Involuntary movements?

Speech

The manner of speaking and its defects are recorded under speech, whereas the content and form of speech are recorded under thought disorders. Does he speak spontaneously or only responds to posed questions? Assess the rate, quantity and flow of speech. It is worthwhile to record a sample of speech for later analysis.

Thought

Inference about the thought process and its disorders are made from the speech sample or the writing sample of the patient. Disorders of form, progression, content and possession may be present. Does the patient have delusions, obsessive ruminations and thought alienation? How does delusion affect his behavior?

Mood and Affect

The patient should be asked about his affective state. Compare the subjective report with what is objectively observed. Is his mood appropriate or not? Congruent or incongruent? Labile? Is the emotional expression blunt? Is the affective expression adequate and appropriate?

Perception

Has the patient any perceptual abnormalities like illusions and hallucinations? If hallucinating, what is the type of hallucination and what is his reaction?

Cognitive Function

Is the patient attentive? Can his attention be easily aroused and sustained? How is his level of concentration? To assess cognitive function some simple tests can be administered. The patient is asked to name the days of the week or names of the month's forwards and backwards. He may be asked to serially subtract 7 or 3 from 100 and spell out the numbers.

Is the patient oriented to time, place and other persons? Orientation to time involves the ability to tell correctly the time of day, date, week, month, year and other related data. Orientation to a place includes correct information of his whereabouts, how he came to be there and other details. Correct identification of people around him ensures orientation to other persons.

Patient's intelligence can be inferred from his conversation and behavior, educational level, vocabulary, ability for abstract thinking and reasoning, general information, etc. Specific tests are used when a more accurate measurement of intelligence is needed. Patient's awareness of his disabilities and readiness for treatment are reflected in insight. Judgment may be inferred from his plans for the future.

PHYSICAL EXAMINATION

A thorough physical examination should be carried out in all cases. It should include body system review, neurological status and laboratory tests.

Particular attention is paid to recent head trauma, episodes of hypertension, changes in personality, speech, or ability to handle activities of daily living. Also note for any movement disorders. Available laboratory data are reviewed for any abnormalities and documented. Particular attention is paid to any abnormalities of hepatic or renal function because these systems metabolize or excrete many psychiatric medications. In addition, abnormal white blood cell and electrolyte levels should be noted.

NEUROLOGICAL EXAMINATION

The purpose of neurological examination is to determine the presence or absence of disease in the nervous system. Nurses are involved in examining the neurological and physical status of the patient as a part of the total physical assessment. The various aspects of neurological examination are as follows:

Levels of Consciousness

Assessment of levels of consciousness includes following categories:
- **Alertness:** Patient is awake, responds immediately and appropriately to all verbal stimuli.
- **Lethargic:** Patient is drowsy and inattentive but arouses easily, frequently goes to sleep.
- **Stuporous:** He arouses with great difficulty and co-operates minimally when stimulated.
- **Semi-comatose:** The patient has lost his ability to respond to verbal stimuli. There is some response to painful stimuli. Little motor function is seen.
- **Comatose:** When the patient is stimulated there is no response to verbal or painful stimuli, no motor activity is seen. Glasgow Coma Scale (GCS) is the most common scoring system used to describe the level of consciousness. Being a standardized method of measuring patient's level of consciousness it eliminates subjectivity and ambiguity. The scale assesses patients according to three aspects of responsiveness—eye-opening, motor, and verbal responses. While a high score of 15 would reflect a fully alert, well oriented person, a score of 3 (the lowest possible score) is indicative of deep coma. A score of 7 or less can be considered as a generally accepted level for coma and indicates the need for a standard of nursing care conducive to the requirement of the comatose patient.

Mental Status Examination

The components of mental status examination are—general appearance, speech, thought process, mood, cognitive functions, attention, concentration, orientation, memory, general knowledge, abstract reasoning, judgment and insight.

Special Cerebral Functions

Assess for agnosia, apraxia and aphasia.
- Agnosia—inability to recognize common objects through the senses
- Apraxia—patient cannot carry out skilled act in the absence of paralysis
- Aphasia—inability to communicate

Cranial Nerve Examination

Cranial nerve (CN) examination provides information about the brainstem and related pathways.
- **Olfactory nerve (CN I):** The function of CN I is purely sensory. Ask the patient to smell and then identify an aromatic, non-irritating odor (coffee, isopropyl alcohol, toothpaste) with each nostril separately and eyes closed. Test with several different odors. If the patient can perceive any one smell, consider the nerve as functioning. Other possible causes of anosmia are cribriform plate fracture, an olfactory bulb or a tract tumor, and previous sinus disorders or surgery.
- **Optic nerve (CN II):** CN II has a purely sensory function. Assessment of the optic nerve involves the following steps:
  - Inspect the eye for foreign bodies, cataracts, inflammation, or other obvious abnormalities.
  - *Test visual acuity:* Have the patient read a newspaper, a sign (from a distance), or a Snellen's chart.
  - Test visual fields to determine whether vision is absent in one or more directions or in a portion of the visual field such as half of the visual field, the middle portion, or both sides. Such losses may indicate various problems and may correlate with the area of the brain involved.
  - Examine the eye fundus with an ophthalmoscope. Gross inspection of the eyes and examination of the fundus can provide information about neurologic disease. Possible causes of abnormal findings include trauma to orbit or eyeball; fracture of optic foramen; diabetic retinopathy; laceration or blood clot in the brain's temporal, parietal, or occipital lobes; and increased ICP.
- **Oculomotor (CN III), trochlear (CN IV) and abducens (CN VI) nerves:** CN III, CN IV and CN VI have only motor components. CN III controls pupil constriction and elevation of the upper lid. Pupils should be equal in size and round.

Approach the pupil from the temporal side while the patient looks straight ahead. Test each pupil for both direct and consensual responses (papillary constriction) to a light. Test accommodation (eyes able to focus on both near and far objects) by having the patient look across the room (away from the light source) and then at your fingers held about 6 inches from the patient's nose.

CN III, CN IV, and CN VI co-ordinate to control eye movements in all six cardinal directions of gaze. Test the function of these nerves by having the patient hold the head still and follow your finger or another object as it is moved in all directions of gaze.

Also observe for nystagmus (involuntary eye movements) seen as fine, rhythmic eye movements that can be vertical, horizontal, or rotational. Possible causes of abnormal findings include: (1) Pressure on CN II, CN IV or CN VI at the brainstem due to fracture of the orbit, (2) increased ICP and (3) tumor at or trauma to the base of the brain.

- **Trigeminal nerve (CN V):** CN V has a motor division and a sensory division. The motor division innervates the muscles of mastication. Test CN V function by asking the patient to clamp the jaws shut, open the mouth against resistance, open the mouth widely, move the jaw from side to side, and make chewing movements. A normal CN V allows all these activities. Document any asymmetry in the temporal muscles. The sensory division mediates all sensations for the entire face, scalp, cornea, and nasal and oral cavities. With the patient's eyes closed, test sensations such as pain (sharp point), touch (wisp of cotton), and temperature (hot and cold metal objects) on both sides of the face from the top of the head (vertex) to the chin.

  Test the corneal reflexes by gently touching the cornea with a sterile wisp of cotton or gently stroking the eye-lash (omit this test during the screening examination). The normal response is brisk eyelid blinking. Possible causes of abnormal findings include a tumor at or trauma to the base of the brain, a fracture of the orbit, and trigeminal neuralgia.

- **Facial nerve (CN VII):** CN VII has both motor division and a sensory division. The motor division innervates muscles controlling facial expression. Observe the face for symmetry and the ability to use facial muscles. Ask the patient to smile, frown, raise the forehead and eyebrows, tightly close the eyes and resist attempts to open them, whistle, show the teeth, and puff out the cheeks. Test the anterior part of the tongue for taste by asking the patient to close the eyes and protrude (stick out) the tongue. Then place a taste substance on one side of the anterior tongue. Have the patient keep the tongue protruded while identifying the taste. Ask the patient to rinse the mouth or drink a small amount of water before testing the other side. Test taste on each side with sweet, salty, acidic or sour (vinegar or lemon) and bitter (coffee) substances.

  Possible causes of abnormal findings are Bell's palsy, temporal bone fracture, and peripheral laceration or contusion of the parotid region.

- **Vestibulocochlear or acoustic nerve (CN VIII):** CN VIII is a sensory nerve with two divisions—cochlear and vestibular. The cochlear nerve permits hearing. Test auditory acuity by having the patient listen to and report on a whispered voice, rustling fingers, or a tuning fork at various distances from the ear. Test bone and air conduction with a tuning fork. The vestibular nerve helps maintain equilibrium by coordinating the muscles of the eye, neck, trunk, and extremities. Equilibrium tests include Romberg's and caloric tests (oculovestibular reflex) and electronystagmography (ENG). Possible causes of abnormal findings include Meniere's syndrome and acoustic neuroma.

- **Glossopharyngeal (CN IX) and vagus (CN X) nerves:** CN IX and CN X have both motor and sensory components. Because of overlapping innervations of the pharynx assess these nerves together. Ask the patient to open the mouth widely and say "Ah". Place a tongue depressor on the first third of the tongue to flatten it and enhance visualization. Observe the position and movement of the uvula and palate. The palate should rise symmetrically with the uvula at the midline. Test the gag reflex by gently touching each side of the pharynx with a tongue depressor which normally elicits a brisk response. Use a small amount of water to assess the ability to swallow. Test the posterior third of the tongue for taste as with CN VII (perform when testing CN VII). Dysfunction of CN IX includes loss of taste and sensation.

  To test the function of CN X ask the patient to cough and to speak. Damage to CN X causes an ineffective cough and a weak, hoarse voice. Possible causes of abnormal findings include brain stem trauma or tumors, neck trauma and stroke.

- **Spinal accessory nerve (CN XI):** CN XI has only a motor component. It innervates the sternocleidomastoid muscle and the upper portion of the trapezius muscle. Ask the patient to (1) elevate the shoulders (with and without resistance), (2) turn (not tilt) the head to one side and then the other, (3) resist attempts to pull the chin back toward the midline and (4) push the head forward against resistance. Disorders may produce drooping of a shoulder, muscle atrophy, weak shoulder shrug, or weak turn of the head. Possible causes of abnormal findings include neck trauma, radical neck surgery, and torticolis.

- **Hypoglossal nerve (CN XII):** CN XII has only a motor component. This nerve innervates the tongue. Ask the patient to open the mouth widely, stick out the tongue, and rapidly move the tongue from side-to-side and, in and out. Document any deviation from midline. Assess strength by having the patient push the tongue against the inside of the cheek while applying external pressure. Possible causes of abnormal findings include neck trauma associated with major blood vessel damage.

Motor Function

Assessment of motor function involves assessing for muscle size, muscle strength, muscle tone, muscle coordination, gait and movement.

- **Muscle size:** Inspect all major muscle groups bilaterally for symmetry, hypertrophy, and atrophy.
- **Muscle strength:** Assess the power in major muscle groups against resistance. Assess and rate muscle strength on a 5-point scale in all four extremities comparing one side with the other as follows:
  - 5/5—normal full strength. Muscle moves actively through the full range of motion against the effects of gravity and applied resistance.
  - 4/5—muscle moves actively through the full range of motion against the effect of gravity with weakness to applied resistance.
  - 3/5—muscle moves actively against the effect of gravity alone.
  - 2/5—muscle moves across a surface but cannot overcome gravity.
  - 1/5—muscle contraction is palpable and visible; trace or flicker movement occurs.
  - 0/5—muscle contraction or movement is undetectable.
- **Muscle tone:** Assess muscle tone while moving each extremity through its range of passive motion. When tone is decreased (hypotonicity) the muscles are soft, flabby, or flaccid; when tone is increased (hypertonicity) the muscles are resistant to movement, rigid, or spastic. Note the presence of abnormal flexion or extension posture.
- **Muscle coordination:** Disorders related to coordination indicate cerebellar or posterior column lesions.
- **Gait and station:** Assess gait and station by having the patient stand still, walk and walk in tandem (one foot in front of the other in a straight line).
- **Movement:** Examine the muscles for fine and gross abnormal movements. Move all the joints through a full range of passive motion. Abnormal findings include pain, joint contractures and muscle resistance.

Sensory Function

Sensory assessment involves testing for touch, pain, vibration, position (proprioception), and discrimination. A complete sensory examination is possible only on a conscious and co-operative patient. Always test sensation with the patient's eyes closed. Help the patient relax and keep warm. Conduct sensory assessment systematically. Test a particular area of the body and then test the corresponding area on the other side.

Abnormalities of Sensation

- **Dysesthesia:** Well localized, irritating sensations such as warmth, cold, itching, tickling, crawling, prickling, and tingling
- **Paresthesia:** Distortions of sensory stimuli (light touch may be experienced as a burning or painful sensation)
- **Anesthesia:** Absence of sense of touch
- **Hypoesthesia:** Reduced sense of touch
- **Hyperesthesia:** Pathologic (abnormal) over perception of touch
- **Analgesia:** Absence of sense of pain
- **Hypoalgesia:** Reduced sense of pain
- **Hyperalgesia:** Increased sense of pain

Assessment of Cerebellar Function

For evaluation of balance and coordination the tests used are:

- **Finger-to-finger test:** It is performed by instructing the patient to place his index finger on the nurse's index finger. He is asked to repeat this for several times in succession on both sides.
- **Finger-to-nose test:** Ask the patient to extend his index finger and then touch the tip of his nose several times in rapid succession. This test is done with patient's eyes both open and closed.
- **Romberg test:** Here the nurse instructs the patient to stand with his feet together with arms positioned at his sides. He is told to close his eyes. This position is maintained for 10 seconds. This test is considered positive only if there is actual loss of balance.
- **Tandem walking test:** This is tested by having the patient assume a normal standing position. He is then instructed to walk over heel on a straight line. Any unsteadiness, lurching or broadening of the gait base is noted.

  Throughout the cerebellar evaluation accuracy of action is assessed during which staggering gait, lack of coordination, tremors are noted as abnormal findings. Abnormalities are usually found in cerebellar diseases such as tumor, multiple sclerosis, motor neuron diseases, etc.

Reflex Activity

Reflex testing evaluates the integrity of specific sensory and motor pathways. Reflex activity assessment which is always a part of neurologic assessment provides information about the nature, location, and progression of neurologic disorders.

Normal Reflexes

Two types of normal reflexes observed are—superficial or cutaneous reflexes and deep tendon or muscle-stretch reflexes.

Superficial (cutaneous) reflexes

These reflexes are elicited by stimulation of the skin or mucous membranes. Stimulus is produced by stroking a sensory zone with an object that will not cause damage. Superficial reflexes [abdominal, plantar, corneal, pharyngeal (gag), cremasteric, and anal] are absent in pyramidal tract disorders, e.g., they are absent on the affected side after a stroke.

- **Abdominal reflex:** Lightly stroking the skin on an abdominal quadrant normally contracts the abdominal muscle thereby moving the umbilicus towards the stimulated side.
- **Plantar reflex:** Scratching the foot's outer aspect of the plantar surface (outer sole) from the heel toward the toes normally contracts or flexes the toes in patients older than 2 years of age.
- **Corneal reflex:** Gently touching the cornea with a wisp of cotton causes reflex blinking. For example, to test the left eye, have the patient look up and to the right and bring the cotton wisp in from the side so that the patient cannot see your hand; then very gently touch the outer edge of the cornea. In an unconscious patient, you can test the corneal reflex by holding the eyelids open and placing a drop of sterile saline on the cornea. This technique prevents inadvertent corneal abrasions.
- **Pharyngeal (gag) reflex:** Gentle stimulation with a tongue blade at the back of the throat and pharynx normally produces gagging. The corneal and pharyngeal reflexes are usually assessed with the cranial nerves as discussed earlier.
- **Cremasteric reflex:** Stroking the inner thigh of a man normally elevates the ipsilateral testicle.
- **Anal reflex:** Stimulate the perianal skin or gently insert a gloved finger into the rectum. Normal response is contraction of the rectal sphincter.

Deep tendon (muscle-stretch) reflexes

Deep tendon reflexes are also called muscle-stretch or myotatic reflexes because reflex muscle contraction normally results from rapid stretching of the muscle. This is produced by sharply striking a muscle tendon's point of insertion with a sudden, brief blow of a reflex hammer. Reflexes commonly assessed include the biceps, triceps, brachioradialis, patella and achilles tendon.

- A biceps jerk (fore arm flexion) is produced by tapping the biceps brachii tendon
- A triceps jerk (fore arm extension) is produced by tapping the triceps brachii tendon at the elbow
- A brachioradial jerk or supinator reflex (elbow flexion, supination of forearm, and flexion of fingers and hand) is produced by taping the styloid process of the radius about 1 to 2 inches above the wrist

- A knee jerk, quadriceps jerk, or patellar reflex (leg extension) is produced by tapping the quadriceps femoris tendon just below the patella
- An ankle jerk (plantiflexion of the foot) is produced by tapping the Achilles tendon

Abnormal Reflexes

Pathologic reflexes indicate neurologic disorders often related to the spinal cord or higher centers. These responses include Babinski's jaw, palm-chin (palmomental), clonus, snout, rooting, sucking, glabella, grasp, and chewing reflexes.

NURSES ROLE IN NEUROLOGICAL EXAMINATION

- Provide a calm, suitable environment
- Collect personal data from the patient and family members
- Set the equipment needed for neurological examination
- Assess the current level of consciousness, monitor vital parameters—temperature, pulse, respiration, blood pressure, pupillary reaction, whether decerebrating or decorticating
- Thorough mental status examination should be done and recorded accurately
- Assessment of cranial nerves should be done correctly and recorded
- Assessment of motor, sensory and cerebellar functions should be done and recorded accurately
- During the examination she should maintain a good support with patient and family members
- She should instruct the procedure correctly and ask the patient to follow it
- Should inform unit doctors of changes, if any

NURSING DIAGNOSIS

Nursing diagnosis is defined as clinical judgments about individual, family or community responses to actual and potential health problems. Nursing diagnoses are used to describe an individual patient's condition, to prescribe nursing interventions, and to delineate the parameters for developing outcome criteria.

A nursing diagnosis statement consists of the problem of patient response and one or more related factors that influence or contribute to the patient's problem or response; signs and symptoms or deficiency characteristics or subjective and objective assessment data that support the nursing diagnosis.

The basic level psychiatric nurse identifies nursing problems using the nomenclature specified by the North American Nursing Diagnoses Association (NANDA).

A nursing diagnosis describes an existing or high-risk problem and requires a three-part statement.
1. Health problem (problem, 'P')
2. Etiological or contributing factors (etiology, 'E')
3. Defining characteristics (signs and symptoms, 'S').

For example:
- High-risk for self-directed violence related to depressed mood, feeling of worthlessness, anger turned inward on the self.
- Powerlessness related to dysfunctional grieving process, lifestyle of helplessness evidenced by feelings of lack of control over life situations, over dependence on others to fulfill needs.

PLANNING

Planning involves setting and prioritizing goals, formulating nursing interventions and developing a care plan in conjunction with the patient based on the nursing diagnoses chosen **(Box 3)**.

Box 3: Effective planning	
• Specific patient needs • Consideration of the patient's strengths and weaknesses	• Encouragement of the patient to help set achievable goals and participate in his own care • Feasible interventions

Nursing interventions with rationales are selected in the planning phase based on patient's identified risk factors and defining characteristics. The process of planning includes:

- Collaboration of the nurse with patients, significant others, and treatment team members
- Identification of priorities of care
- Critical decisions regarding the use of psychotherapeutic principles and practices (Identify the most appropriate nursing intervention)
- Coordination and delegation of responsibilities.

In this, the nurse will choose nursing interventions appropriate to an individual's identified problem with specific expected outcomes.

Once the nursing diagnoses are identified, the next step is the prioritization of the problems in the order of importance. Highest priority is given to those problems that are life-threatening. Next in the priority are those problems that are likely to cause destructive changes. Lowest in priority are those issues that are related to normative or developmental experiences. Psychiatric nurses often use Maslow's hierarchy of needs to prioritize nursing diagnosis.

Outcome Identification

Outcomes can be defined as a patient's response to the care received. Outcomes are the end result of the process. Measuring outcomes not only demonstrates clinical effectiveness but also helps to promote rational clinical decision-making on the part of the nurse. Each outcome must follow certain criteria **(Box 4)**.

Box 4: Criteria for effective outcome identification	
• Relate directly to the nursing diagnosis • Be measurable, time limited, and realistic • Be stated as a desired patient outcome of nursing care	• Reflect the desires of the patient and his family • Be stated in a way that the patient and his family can understand

Diagnosis	Outcome	Intervention
Impaired social interaction (isolates self from others)	Patient will attend group sessions everyday	Using a contract format explain the role and responsibility of patients

Correct and Incorrect Outcome Statement

Nursing diagnosis	Correct outcome	Incorrect outcome
Anxiety	Verbalizes feeling calm, relaxed, with absence of muscle tension and diaphoresis; practices deep breathing	Exhibits decreased anxiety, engages in stress reduction
Ineffective coping	Makes own decisions to attend groups; seeks staff for interaction	Demonstrates effective coping abilities

▌ IMPLEMENTATION

In the implementation phase, the nurse sets interventions prescribed in the planning phase.

Nursing interventions (also known as nursing orders or nursing prescriptions) are the most powerful pieces of the nursing process. Interventions are selected to achieve patient outcome and to prevent or reduce problems. Implementation serves as a blueprint of plan.

Nursing interventions are classified as independent, interdependent and dependent.

Nursing Intervention in Psychiatric Nursing

Interventions for Biological Dimension

- Self-care activities
- Activity and exercise
- Nutritional intervention
- Hydration intervention

- Thermoregulation intervention
- Pain management
- Medication management

Interventions for Psychological Dimension

- Counseling intervention
- Conflict resolution
- Bibliotherapy
- Reminiscence therapy
- Relaxation intervention
- Behavior therapy
- Cognitive therapy
- Psychoeducation
- Spiritual intervention

Interventions for Social Dimension

- Group intervention
- Family intervention
- Milieu therapy

EVALUATION

Evaluation is the process of determining the value of an intervention. Nurses determine the effectiveness of interventions with particular patients. Nurses evaluate selected interventions by judging the patient's progress towards the outcome set down in the nursing care plan.

PRACTICE COMPETENCIES

On completion of the course, the students will be able to:
- Assess patients with mental health problems/disorders
- Observe and assist in various treatment modalities or therapies
- Counsel and educate patients and families
- Perform individual and group psychoeducation
- Provide nursing care to patients with mental health problems/disorders
- Motivate patients in the community for early treatment and follow-up
- Observe the assessment and care of patients with substance abuse disorders in de-addiction center

Assignments

- **Assignment 1:** Philosophy, Objectives and Physical Set-up of the Mental Hospital/Nursing Home/Institution
- **Assignment 2:** History Taking and Mental Status Examination in Psychiatric Nursing - I
- **Assignment 3:** History Taking and Mental Status Examination in Psychiatric Nursing - II
- **Assignment 4:** Psychometric Assessment Report
- **Assignment 5:** Neurological Examination
- **Assignment 6:** Health Education
- **Assignment 7:** Observational Report on Outpatient Department
- **Assignment 8:** Nursing Care Plan for Child with Psychiatric Disorder
- **Assignment 9:** Observational Report on Child Guidance Clinic
- **Assignment 10:** Case Study
- **Assignment 11:** Nursing Care Plan for Patient with Psychiatric Disorder - I
- **Assignment 12:** Nursing Care Plan for Patient with Psychiatric Disorder - II
- **Assignment 13:** Nursing Care Plan for Patient with Psychiatric Disorder - III
- **Assignment 14:** Clinical/Case Presentation
- **Assignment 15:** Process Recording - I
- **Assignment 16:** Process Recording - II
- **Assignment 17:** Administration of Psychotropic Drugs - I
- **Assignment 18:** Administration of Psychotropic Drugs - II
- **Assignment 19:** Administration of Psychotropic Drugs - III
- **Assignment 20:** Assist the Patient for Electroconvulsive Therapy
- **Assignment 21:** Assist the Patient for Individual Psychotherapy
- **Assignment 22:** Assist the Patient for Family Psychotherapy
- **Assignment 23:** Assist the Patient for Group Psychotherapy
- **Assignment 24:** Assist the Patient for Occupational Psychotherapy
- **Assignment 25:** Assist the Patient for Behavioral Psychotherapy
- **Assignment 26:** Assist the Patient for Recreational Therapy
- **Assignment 27:** Assist the Patient for Play Therapy
- **Assignment 28:** Preparation of Patients for Activities of Daily Living - I
- **Assignment 29:** Preparation of Patients for Activities of Daily Living - II
- **Assignment 30:** Preparation of Patients for Activities of Daily Living - III
- **Assignment 31:** Admission Procedure
- **Assignment 32:** Discharge Procedure
- **Assignment 33:** Health Education
- **Assignment 34:** Psychotropic Drug Book
- **Assignment 35:** Community Case Work
- **Assignment 36:** Observational Report on Field Visits
- **Assignment 37:** Observational Report on De-addiction Center

ASSIGNMENT - 1

Philosophy, Objectives and Physical Set-up of the Mental Hospital/Nursing Home/Institution

Philosophy of Mental Hospital/Nursing Home

Objectives

1.

2.

3.

4.

5.

Physical Set-up of the Mental Hospital/Nursing Home/Institution

ASSIGNMENT - 2

History Taking and Mental Status Examination in Psychiatric Nursing - I

I. Identification Data

Name: Age: Sex:

Name of the Father/Spouse: Education: Occupation:

Income: Marital Status: Religion:

Address: Mobile No.:   Aadhar No.:

Informant:

Information: Relevant/Irrelevant, Adequate/Inadequate

II. Presenting Chief Complaint

(With duration in chronological order, in patient's and informant's own words)

III. History of Present Illness

Duration (days/weeks/months/years):

Mode of onset:

Course:

Intensity:

Precipitating factors: Yes/No, if yes, explain

Description of present illness: Chronological description of abnormal behavior, start with early symptoms and explain duration, context, frequency, increasing factors, decreasing factors, outcome of those symptoms, associated problems like suicide, homicide, disruptive behavior; thought content, speech, mood states, abnormal perception, biological functioning (sleep, appetite, libido, hygiene, bowel and bladder habits), social functioning (interaction with family members, friends, relatives and neighbors), occupational functioning (functioning, absenteeism, pending enquiry), changes in ADLs.

IV. Negative History

V. Medical Illness

VI. Past Psychiatric and Medical History

VII. Family History

Name of the family member	Age	Education	Occupation	Health status	Relationship with the patient	Age at death and mode of death

Genogram (family of origin, three generations):

VIII. Personal History

a. Perinatal history

b. Childhood history

c. Educational history

d. Play history

e. Emotional problems during adolescence

f. Puberty

g. Obstetrical history

h. Occupational history

i. Sexual and martial history

j. Premorbid personality

Mental Status Examination

a. General Appearance and Behavior

Appearance:

Facial expression:

Level of grooming:

Level of cleanliness:

Level of consciousness:

Mode of entry:

Behavior:

Cooperativeness:

Eye-to-eye contact:

Psychomotor activity:

Rapport:

Gesturing:

Posturing:

Other movements:

Other catatonic phenomena:

Conversion and dissociative signs:

Compulsive acts or rituals or habits:

Hallucinatory behavior:

b. Speech

Initiation:

Reaction time:

Rate:

Productivity:

Volume:

Tone:

Relevance:

Stream (flow and rhythm of speech):

Coherence:

Others:

Sample of speech (in response to open-ended questions, verbatim in 2 or 3 sentences):

c. Mood and Affect

Subjective report:

Objective assessment:

Predominant mood state:

Congruent to the thought process:

Lability:

d. Thought

Stream (flow of thought):

Form (formal thought disorder):

Possession:

Content:

e. Perception

Illusions:

Hallucinations:

Somatic passivity:

Déjà vu/jamais vu:

Depersonalization/derealization:

f. Cognitive Function (Neuropsychiatric Assessment)

Consciousness:

Orientation:

Attention:

Concentration:

Memory

Immediate:

Recent:

Remote:

Intelligence:

Abstraction:

Judgment:

g. Insight

Treatment:

Diagnostic Formulation

Name and Signature of the Student   **Name and Signature of the Supervisor**

Proforma for Evaluating History Collection in Psychiatric Nursing - I

S. No.	Criteria	Max. marks	Marks obtained
1.	Bio-data of the patient	1	
2.	Chief complaints	2	
3.	History of present illness	5	
4.	Past history	2	
5.	Personal history	2	
6.	Premorbid personality	3	
7.	Physical examination	5	
	Total	**20**	

Remarks:

Signature of the Student   **Signature of the Supervisor**

Proforma for Evaluating Mental Status Examination in Psychiatric Nursing - I

S. No.	Criteria	Max. marks	Marks obtained
1.	General appearance and behavior	½	
2.	Speech	½	
3.	Mood	½	
4.	Thought	1	
5.	Perception	1	
6.	Cognitive function		
	• Orientation	½	
	• Attention and concentration	½	
	• Memory	1	
	• Intelligence and general information	1	
	• Abstract thinking	1	
7.	Judgment	½	
8.	Insight	1	
9.	Summary	1	
	Total	**10**	

Remarks:

Signature of the Student   **Signature of the Supervisor**

ASSIGNMENT - 3

History Taking and Mental Status Examination in Psychiatric Nursing - II

I. Identification Data

Name: Age: Sex:

Name of the Father/Spouse: Education: Occupation:

Income: Marital Status: Religion:

Address: Mobile No.:   Aadhar No.:

Informant:

Information: Relevant/Irrelevant, Adequate/Inadequate

II. Presenting Chief Complaint

(With duration in chronological order, in patient's and informant's own words)

III. History of Present Illness

Duration (days/weeks/months/years):
Mode of onset:
Course:
Intensity:
Precipitating factors: Yes/No, if yes, explain

Description of present illness: Chronological description of abnormal behavior, start with the early symptoms and explain duration, context, frequency, increasing factors, decreasing factors, outcome of those symptoms, associated problems like suicide, homicide, disruptive behavior; thought content, speech, mood states, abnormal perception, biological functioning (sleep, appetite, libido, hygiene, bowel and bladder habits), social functioning (interaction with family members, friends, relatives and neighbors), occupational functioning (functioning, absenteeism, pending enquiry), changes in ADLs.

IV. Negative History

V. Medical Illness

VI. Past Psychiatric and Medical History

VII. Family History

Name of the family member	Age	Education	Occupation	Health status	Relationship with the patient	Age at death and mode of death

Genogram (family of origin, three generations):

VIII. Personal History

a. Perinatal history

b. Childhood history

c. Educational history

d. Play history

e. Emotional problems during adolescence

f. Puberty

g. Obstetrical history

h. Occupational history

i. Sexual and martial history

j. Premorbid personality

Mental Status Examination

a. General Appearance and Behavior

Appearance:

Facial expression:

Level of grooming:

Level of cleanliness:

Level of consciousness:

Mode of entry:

Behavior:

Cooperativeness:

Eye-to-eye contact:

Psychomotor activity:

Rapport:

Gesturing:

Posturing:

Other movements:

Other catatonic phenomena:

Conversion and dissociative signs:

Compulsive acts or rituals or habits:

Hallucinatory behavior:

b. Speech

Initiation:

Reaction time:

Rate:

Productivity:

Volume:

Tone:

Relevance:

Stream (flow and rhythm of speech):

Coherence:

Others:

Sample of speech (in response to open-ended questions, verbatim in 2 or 3 sentences):

c. Mood and Affect

Subjective report:

Objective assessment:

Predominant mood state:

Congruent to the thought process:

Lability:

d. Thought

Stream (flow of thought):

Form (formal thought disorder):

Possession:

Content:

e. Perception

Illusions:

Hallucinations:

Somatic passivity:

Déjà vu/jamais vu:

Depersonalization/derealization:

f. Cognitive Function (Neuropsychiatric Assessment)

Consciousness:

Orientation:

Attention:

Concentration:

Memory

Immediate:

Recent:

Remote:

Intelligence:

Abstraction:

Judgment:

g. Insight

Treatment:

Diagnostic Formulation

Name and Signature of the Student   **Name and Signature of the Supervisor**

Proforma for Evaluating History Collection in Psychiatric Nursing - II

S. No.	Criteria	Max. marks	Marks obtained
1.	Bio-data of the patient	1	
2.	Chief complaints	2	
3.	History of present illness	5	
4.	Past history	2	
5.	Personal history	2	
6.	Premorbid personality	3	
7.	Physical examination	5	
	Total	**20**	

Remarks:

Signature of the Student　　　　　　　　　　　　　　　　**Signature of the Supervisor**

Proforma for Evaluating Mental Status Examination in Psychiatric Nursing - II

S. No.	Criteria	Max. marks	Marks obtained
1.	General appearance and behavior	½	
2.	Speech	½	
3.	Mood	½	
4.	Thought	1	
5.	Perception	1	
6.	Cognitive function		
	♦ Orientation	½	
	♦ Attention and concentration	½	
	♦ Memory	1	
	♦ Intelligence and general information	1	
	♦ Abstract thinking	1	
7.	Judgment	½	
8.	Insight	1	
9.	Summary	1	
	Total	**10**	

Remarks:

Signature of the Student　　　　　　　　　　　　　　　　**Signature of the Supervisor**

ASSIGNMENT - 4

Psychometric Assessment Report

Demographic Data

Name of the patient: Age: Sex:

Religion: IP No.:   Marital Status:

Education: Occupation:

Address:

Diagnosis:

Name of the psychological test:

Indications for assessment:

Preparation of the patient:

Description of the test:

Result/score of the test:

Signature of the Student   **Signature of the Supervisor**

ASSIGNMENT - 5

Neurological Examination

I. Level of Consciousness

Alert/lethargic/stuporous/semi-comatose/comatose

Score of Glasgow coma scale:

II. Mental Status Examination

General appearance:

Speech:

Thought process:

Mood:

Cognitive functions

- Attention and concentration
    - Digit span—backward, forward
    - Serial 7
- Orientation
    - Time
    - Place
    - Person
- Memory
    - Immediate
    - Recent
    - Remote
- General knowledge
- Abstract reasoning
- Judgment
- Insight

III. Special Cerebral Functions

Agnosia/apraxia/aphasia

IV. Cranial Nerve Examination

Olfactory nerve: Sense of smell—present/absent

Optic nerve: Inspection of eye—inflammation/cataract/foreign bodies/any abnormalities
- Visual acuity (Snellen's chart)
- Visual field examination
  - Right eye
  - Left eye
- Ophthalmoscope examination
- Color vision—present/absent

Oculomotor, trochlear and abducent nerves
- Pupillary reaction to light—reacting/not reacting
- Pupillary size—equal/unequal
- Eye movement in six directions—normal/abnormal
- Nystagmus—present/absent
- Diplopia—present/absent

Trigeminal nerve
- Corneal reflex—present/absent
- Facial sensory response—present/absent
- Mandibular strength—adequate/hypotonia

Facial nerve
- Facial expressions—normal/hypotonia
- Taste sensation—present/absent

Vestibule cochlear nerve
- Auditory acuity test
- Air conduction
- Bone conduction

Glossopharyngeal and vagus nerve
- Gag reflex—present/absent
- Swallowing reflex—present/absent
- Position and movement of uvula and palate—normal position/deviation
- Sensation of taste—present/absent

Spinal accessory nerve
- Sternocleidomastoid muscle strength—normal/hypotonia
- Elevation of shoulders—adequate strength/weakness
- Turning of head—adequate/inadequate

Hypoglossal nerve
- Tongue movement—normal/abnormal

V. Motor Function Assessment

- Muscle size
- Muscle strength
- Muscle tone
- Muscle coordination
- Gait
- Movements of all the joints
- Deformities
- Abnormal movements

VI. Sensory Function Assessment

- Pain sensation—present/absent
- Temperature sensation—present/absent
- Touch sensation—present/absent
- Vibration sensation—present/absent

VII. Assessment of Cerebellar Function

- Finger to finger test—normal/abnormal
- Finger to nose test—normal/abnormal
- Romberg test—normal/unable to perform
- Tandem walking test—normal/unable to perform

VIII. Assessment of Reflexes

- Superficial reflexes—present/absent
- Abdominal/plantar/corneal/pharyngeal/cremasteric/anal
- Deep tendon reflexes—present/absent
- Biceps/triceps/brachioradial/patellar/achilles
- Any abnormal reflexes—present/absent

IX. Summary

Signature of the Student   **Signature of the Supervisor**

ASSIGNMENT - 6

Health Education

Name of the topic:

Group and number:

Place:

Date and time:

Duration of health education:

Name of the student:

Name of the supervisor:

Method of teaching:

AV aids:

General objectives:

Specific objectives:

Specific objective	Content	AV aids	Evaluation

Specific objective	Content	AV aids	Evaluation

Specific objective	Content	AV aids	Evaluation

Specific objective	Content	AV aids	Evaluation

References:

Name and Signature of the Student   **Name and Signature of the Supervisor**

ASSIGNMENT - 7

Observational Report on Outpatient Department

Duration of posting from .... to ....

Name of the hospital and address:

Average number of patients visit OPD per month:

List common psychiatric conditions which you observed in OPD:

List various services provided in the OPD:

Give a brief account of the learning experiences achieved from the OPD posting:

Describe the physical set-up of the OPD:

Name and Signature of the Student   **Name and Signature of the Supervisor**

ASSIGNMENT - 8

Nursing Care Plan for Child with Psychiatric Disorder

A. Demographic Data

Name: Age: Sex:

Address:

Income: Residence: Urban/Semi-urban/Rural

Hospital No.:

Informant: Mother/Father/Others

B. Chief Complaints (With Duration in Brief)

C. History of Present Illness

D. Family History

Nuclear/non-nuclear

Consanguineous marriage/non-consanguineous marriage

History of mental illness/epilepsy/mentally retarded/any other

Genogram (three generations):

E. Personal History

Antenatal history:

Perinatal history:

Postnatal history:

Milestones:

Current schooling:

Habits:

Interest and talents:

Sexual history:

F. Past History

Psychiatric:

Neurotic:

Others:

G. Current Functioning

1. Intelligence: Above average/average/below average

2. School performance: Above average/average/below average

3. Self-help skills (age appropriate)

    a. Toilet: Yes/No

    b. Dressing: Yes/No

    c. Eating: Yes/No

    d. Bathing/washing: Yes/No

H. Schooling History

1. Age at starting schooling

2. Academic performance

3. School refusal

I. Menstrual and Sexual History

1. Body image concern

2. Menstrual history

J. Temperament History

1. Activity level

2. Adaptability to environment

3. Impulsivity

4. Regularity in biological function

5. Intensity of reaction

6. Quality of mood

7. Shy, fearful and anxious of certain places: Yes/No

8. Excessive tantrums: Yes/No

9. Excessive clinging behavior: Yes/No

K. Physical Examination

Vision

Hearing

CNS

Respiratory system

Cardiovascular system

Gastrointestinal system

Genitourinary system

L. Treatment History till Date

M. Mental Status Examination

Attention and concentration

Activity level

Motor behavior

Speech and language ability

General intelligence

Mood and affect

Thought processes

Perception

Summary

Nursing Management

Nursing Assessment

Objective data:

Subjective data:

List of nursing diagnoses:

Nursing Care Plan

Assessment	Nursing diagnosis	Goal/objective	Intervention

Implementation	Rationale	Evaluation

Assessment	Nursing diagnosis	Goal/objective	Intervention

Implementation	Rationale	Evaluation

Medications

S. No.	Name of the drug	Dose and route	Mechanism of action	Adverse effects	Nurse's responsibility

Health education:

Conclusion:

Name and Signature of the Student   **Name and Signature of the Supervisor**

ASSIGNMENT - 9

Observational Report on Child Guidance Clinic

Date of visit :

Describe philosophy of the child guidance clinic:

List the objectives of clinic:

1.

2.

3.

4.

5.

List various services provided by the clinic:

1.

2.

3.

4.

Draw the organizational structure of the clinic:

Briefly describe the physical set-up:

Describe staffing pattern and duty timings of the staff:

Mention admission procedure:

Give a brief account of learning experience achieved from this visit:

Name and Signature of the Student   **Name and Signature of the Supervisor**

ASSIGNMENT - 10

Case Study

Identification Data

Name: Age: Sex:

Name of the Father/Spouse:

Address:

Education: Occupation: Income:

Marital Status: Religion:

Informant:

Information: Relevant/Irrelevant, Adequate/Inadequate

Presenting Chief Complaint

(With duration in chronological order, in patient's own words and informant's own words)

History of Present Illness

Duration:

Mode of onset:

Course:

Intensity:

Precipitating factors:

Description of present illness:
While describing present illness consider chronological description of abnormal behavior, associated problems like suicide, homicide, disruptive behavior; thought content, speech, mood states, abnormal perception, biological functioning, social functioning, occupational functioning, changes in ADLs

Past Psychiatric and Medical History

Family History

Name of the family member	Age	Education	Occupation	Health status	Health status relationship with the patient	Age at death and mode of death

Genogram (family of origin, three generations):

Personal History

A. Perinatal History

B. Childhood History

C. Educational History

D. Play History

E. Emotional Problems during Adolescence

F. Puberty

G. Obstetrical History

H. Occupational History

I. Sexual and Marital History

J. Premorbid Personality

Mental Status Examination

A. *General Appearance and Behavior*

Appearance:

Facial expression:

Level of grooming:

Level of cleanliness:

Level of consciousness:

Mode of entry:

Behavior:

Cooperativeness:

Eye-to-eye contact:

Psychomotor activity:

Rapport:

Gesturing:

Posturing:

Other movements:

Other catatonic phenomena:

Conversion and dissociative signs:

Hallucinatory behavior:

B. *Speech*

Initiation:

Reaction time:

Rate:

Productivity:

Volume:

Tone:

Relevance:

Stream (flow and rhythm of speech):

Coherence:

Others:

Sample of speech (in response to open-ended questions, verbatim in 2 or 3 sentences):

C. *Mood and Affect*

Subjective:

Objective:

Predominant mood state:

D. *Thought*

Stream (flow of thought):

Form (formal thought disorder):

Content:

E. *Perception*

Illusions:

Hallucinations (specify type and give example):

Somatic passivity:

Déjà vu/jamais vu:

Depersonalization/derealization:

F. *Cognitive Function (Neuropsychiatric Assessment)*

Consciousness:

Orientation:

- Time:

- Place:

- Person:

Attention:

Concentration:

Memory

- Immediate:

- Recent:

- Remote:

Intelligence

Abstraction

Judgment

G. *Insight*

Diagnostic Formulation

Physical Examination

General examination:

Temperature:

Pulse:

Respiration:

Blood pressure (BP):

CVS, peripheral pulsations:

Respiratory system:

Gastrointestinal:

Musculoskeletal system:

Lymph nodes:

Breasts:

Pelvic examination:

Any other signs:

Summary:

Investigations

Name of the investigation	Patient value	Normal value	Remarks

Book Picture of Disease Condition

Introduction

Definition

Incidence

Etiology

Book picture	Patient picture

Psychopathology

Clinical Manifestations

Book picture	Patient picture

Investigations and Diagnosis

Book picture	Patient picture

Treatment (psychopharmacological and psychosocial management)

Book picture	Patient picture

Nursing Management

Nursing Assessment

Objective data:

Subjective data:

List of nursing diagnoses:

Nursing Care Plan

Assessment	Nursing diagnosis	Goal/objective	Intervention

Implementation	Rationale	Evaluation

Assessment	Nursing diagnosis	Goal/objective	Intervention

Implementation	Rationale	Evaluation

Medications

S. No.	Name of the drug	Dose and route	Mechanism of action	Adverse effects	Nurse's responsibility

Health education:

Conclusion:

References:

Name and Signature of the Student   **Name and Signature of the Supervisor**

Proforma for Evaluating Case Study in Psychiatric Nursing

Name of the student: Name of the patient:

Year: Hospital No.:

Register No.:   Age:

Area/ward: Sex:

Date of submission: Diagnosis:

S. No.	Criteria	Max. marks	Marks obtained
1.	History taking	2	
2.	Mental status examination	2	
3.	Description of diseased condition		
	◆ Definition	1	
	◆ Etiological factors	1	
	◆ Clinical manifestations (according to book and patient)	2	
4.	Diagnosis	1	
5.	Prognosis	1	
6.	Management		
	◆ Pharmacological therapy	1	
	◆ Psychological therapies	1	
	◆ Rehabilitation (according to book and patient)	1	
7.	Nursing Management		
	◆ Nursing assessment	½	
	◆ Nursing diagnosis	1	
	◆ Planning	½	
	◆ Implementation	3	
	◆ Evaluation	½	
	◆ Health education	1	
8.	Bibliography	½	
	Total	**20**	

Remarks:

Signature of the Student   **Signature of the Supervisor**

ASSIGNMENT - 11

Nursing Care Plan for Patient with Psychiatric Disorder - I

Identification Data

Name: Age: Sex:

Name of the Father/Spouse:

Address:

Education: Occupation: Income:

Marital Status: Religion:

Informant:

Information: Relevant/Irrelevant, Adequate/Inadequate

Presenting Chief Complaint

(With duration in chronological order, in patient's own words and informant's own words)

History of Present Illness

Duration:

Mode of onset:

Course:

Intensity:

Precipitating factors:

Description of present illness:
While describing present illness consider chronological description of abnormal behavior, associated problems like suicide, homicide, disruptive behavior; thought content, speech, mood states, abnormal perception, biological functioning, social functioning, occupational functioning, changes in ADLs.

Past Psychiatric and Medical History

Family History

Name of the family member	Age	Education	Occupation	Health status	Relationship with the patient	Age at death and mode of death

Genogram (family of origin, three generations):

Personal History

A. Perinatal History

B. Childhood History

C. Educational History

D. Play History

E. Emotional Problems during Adolescence

F. Puberty

G. Obstetrical History

H. Occupational History

I. Sexual and Marital History

J. Premorbid Personality

Mental Status Examination

A. *General Appearance and Behavior*

Appearance:

Facial expression:

Level of grooming:

Level of cleanliness:

Level of consciousness:

Mode of entry:

Behavior:

Cooperativeness:

Eye-to-eye contact:

Psychomotor activity:

Rapport:

Gesturing:

Posturing:

Other movements:

Other catatonic phenomena:

Conversion and dissociative signs:

Hallucinatory behavior:

B. *Speech*

Initiation:

Reaction time:

Rate:

Productivity:

Volume:

Tone:

Relevance:

Stream (flow and rhythm of speech):

Coherence:

Others:

Sample of speech (in response to open-ended questions, verbatim in 2 or 3 sentences):

C. Mood and Affect

Subjective:

Objective:

Predominant mood state:

D. Thought

Stream (flow of thought):

Form (formal thought disorder):

Content:

E. Perception

Illusions:

Hallucinations (specify type and give example):

Somatic passivity:

Déjà vu/jamais vu:

Depersonalization/derealization:

F. Cognitive Function (Neuropsychiatric Assessment)

Consciousness:

Orientation:

- Time:

- Place:

- Person:

Attention:

- Digit forward:

- Digit backward:

Concentration:

Memory

- Immediate:

- Recent:

- Remote:

Intelligence

Abstraction

Judgment

G. *Insight*

Diagnostic Formulation

Physical Examination

General examination:

Temperature:

Pulse:

Respiration:

Blood pressure (BP):

CVS, peripheral pulsations:

Respiratory system:

Gastrointestinal:

Musculoskeletal system:

Lymph nodes:

Breasts:

Pelvic examination:

Any other signs:

Summary:

Investigations

Name of the investigation	Patient value	Normal value	Remarks

Nursing Management

Nursing Assessment

Objective data:

Subjective data:

List of nursing diagnoses:

Nursing Care Plan

Assessment	Nursing diagnosis	Goal/objective	Intervention

Implementation	Rationale	Evaluation

Assessment	Nursing diagnosis	Goal/objective	Intervention

Implementation	Rationale	Evaluation

Medications

S. No.	Name of the drug	Dose and route	Mechanism of action	Adverse effects	Nurse's responsibility

Health education:

Conclusion:

Name and Signature of the Student   **Name and Signature of the Supervisor**

Proforma for Evaluating Care Plan in Psychiatric Nursing

Name of the student: Name of the patient:

Year: Hospital No.:

Register No.:   Age:

Area/ward: Sex:

Date of submission: Diagnosis:

S. No.	Criteria	Max. marks	Marks obtained
1.	Bio-data of the patient	½	
2.	Chief complaints	½	
3.	History of present illness	1	
4.	Past history	½	
5.	Personal history	1	
6.	Premorbid personality	½	
7.	Physical examination	1	
8.	Mental status examination	3	
9.	Nursing assessment data:		
	◆ Objective	½	
	◆ Subjective	½	
10.	Nursing diagnoses	2	
11.	Short-term goals and long-term goals	1	
12.	Plan of action with rationale	2	
13.	Implementation	2	
14.	Evaluation	1	
15.	Health education	2	
16.	Progress notes	1	
	Total	**20**	

Remarks:

Signature of the Student   **Signature of the Supervisor**

ASSIGNMENT - 12

Nursing Care Plan for Patient with Psychiatric Disorder - II

Identification Data

Name: Age: Sex:

Name of the Father/Spouse:

Address:

Education: Occupation: Income:

Marital Status: Religion:

Informant:

Information: Relevant/Irrelevant, Adequate/Inadequate

Presenting Chief Complaint

(With duration in chronological order, in patient's own words and informant's own words)

History of Present Illness

Duration:

Mode of onset:

Course:

Intensity:

Precipitating factors:

Description of present illness:
While describing present illness consider chronological description of abnormal behavior, associated problems like suicide, homicide, disruptive behavior; thought content, speech, mood states, abnormal perception, biological functioning, social functioning, occupational functioning, changes in ADLs.

Past Psychiatric and Medical History

Family History

Name of the family member	Age	Education	Occupation	Health status	Relationship with the patient	Age at death and mode of death

Genogram (family of origin, three generations):

Personal History

A. Perinatal History

B. Childhood History

C. Educational History

D. Play History

E. Emotional Problems during Adolescence

F. Puberty

G. Obstetrical History

H. Occupational History

I. Sexual and Marital History

J. Premorbid Personality

Mental Status Examination

A. *General Appearance and Behavior*

Appearance:

Facial expression:

Level of grooming:

Level of cleanliness:

Level of consciousness:

Mode of entry:

Behavior:

Cooperativeness:

Eye-to-eye contact:

Psychomotor activity:

Rapport:

Gesturing:

Posturing:

Other movements:

Other catatonic phenomena:

Conversion and dissociative signs:

Hallucinatory behavior:

B. *Speech*

Initiation:

Reaction time:

Rate:

Productivity:

Volume:

Tone:

Relevance:

Stream (flow and rhythm of speech):

Coherence:

Others:

Sample of speech (in response to open-ended questions, verbatim in 2 or 3 sentences):

C. Mood and Affect

Subjective:

Objective:

Predominant mood state:

D. Thought

Stream (flow of thought):

Form (formal thought disorder):

Content:

E. Perception

Illusions:

Hallucinations (specify type and give example):

Somatic passivity:

Déjà vu/jamais vu:

Depersonalization/derealization:

F. Cognitive Function (Neuropsychiatric Assessment)

Consciousness:

Orientation:

- Time:

- Place:

- Person:

Attention:

- Digit forward:

- Digit backward:

Concentration:

Memory

- Immediate:

- Recent:

- Remote:

Intelligence

Abstraction

Judgment

G. Insight

Diagnostic Formulation

Physical Examination

General examination:

Temperature:

Pulse:

Respiration:

Blood pressure (BP):

CVS, peripheral pulsations:

Respiratory system:

Gastrointestinal:

Musculoskeletal system:

Lymph nodes:

Breasts:

Pelvic examination:

Any other signs:

Summary:

Investigations

Name of the investigation	Patient value	Normal value	Remarks

Nursing Management

Nursing Assessment

Objective data:

Subjective data:

List of nursing diagnoses:

Nursing Care Plan

Assessment	Nursing diagnosis	Goal/objective	Intervention

Nursing Care Plan

Implementation	Rationale	Evaluation

Assessment	Nursing diagnosis	Goal/objective	Intervention

Implementation	Rationale	Evaluation

Medications

S. No.	Name of the drug	Dose and route	Mechanism of action	Adverse effects	Nurse's responsibility

Health education:

Conclusion:

Name and Signature of the Student **Name and Signature of the Supervisor**

Proforma for Evaluating Care Plan in Psychiatric Nursing

Name of the student: Name of the patient:

Year: Hospital No.:

Register No.:   Age:

Area/ward: Sex:

Date of submission: Diagnosis:

S. No.	Criteria	Max. marks	Marks obtained
1.	Bio-data of the patient	½	
2.	Chief complaints	½	
3.	History of present illness	1	
4.	Past history	½	
5.	Personal history	1	
6.	Premorbid personality	½	
7.	Physical examination	1	
8.	Mental status examination	3	
9.	Nursing assessment data:		
	• Objective	½	
	• Subjective	½	
10.	Nursing diagnoses	2	
11.	Short-term goals and long-term goals	1	
12.	Plan of action with rationale	2	
13.	Implementation	2	
14.	Evaluation	1	
15.	Health education	2	
16.	Progress notes	1	
	Total	**20**	

Remarks:

Signature of the Student   **Signature of the Supervisor**

ASSIGNMENT - 13

Nursing Care Plan for Patient with Psychiatric Disorder - III

Identification Data

Name: Age: Sex:

Name of the Father/Spouse:

Address:

Education: Occupation: Income:

Marital Status: Religion:

Informant:

Information: Relevant/Irrelevant, Adequate/Inadequate

Presenting Chief Complaint

(With duration in chronological order, in patient's own words and informant's own words)

History of Present Illness

Duration:

Mode of onset:

Course:

Intensity:

Precipitating factors:

Description of present illness:
While describing present illness consider chronological description of abnormal behavior, associated problems like suicide, homicide, disruptive behavior; thought content, speech, mood states, abnormal perception, biological functioning, social functioning, occupational functioning, changes in ADLs.

Past Psychiatric and Medical History

Family History

Name of the family member	Age	Education	Occupation	Health status	Relationship with the patient	Age at death and mode of death

Genogram (family of origin, three generations):

Personal History

A. Perinatal History

B. Childhood History

C. Educational History

D. Play History

E. Emotional Problems during Adolescence

F. Puberty

G. Obstetrical History

H. Occupational History

I. Sexual and Marital History

J. Premorbid Personality

Mental Status Examination

A. *General Appearance and Behavior*

Appearance:

Facial expression:

Level of grooming:

Level of cleanliness:

Level of consciousness:

Mode of entry:

Behavior:

Cooperativeness:

Eye-to-eye contact:

Psychomotor activity:

Rapport:

Gesturing:

Posturing:

Other movements:

Other catatonic phenomena:

Conversion and dissociative signs:

Hallucinatory behavior:

B. *Speech*

Initiation:

Reaction time:

Rate:

Productivity:

Volume:

Tone:

Relevance:

Stream (flow and rhythm of speech):

Coherence:

Others:

Sample of speech (in response to open-ended questions, verbatim in 2 or 3 sentences):

C. Mood and Affect

Subjective:

Objective:

Predominant mood state:

D. Thought

Stream (flow of thought):

Form (formal thought disorder):

Content:

E. Perception

Illusions:

Hallucinations (specify type and give example):

Somatic passivity:

Déjà vu/jamais vu:

Depersonalization/derealization:

F. Cognitive Function (Neuropsychiatric Assessment)

Consciousness:

Orientation:

- Time:

- Place:

- Person:

Attention:

- Digit forward:

- Digit backward:

Concentration:

Memory

- Immediate:

- Recent:

- Remote:

Intelligence

Abstraction

Judgment

G. Insight

Diagnostic Formulation

Physical Examination

General examination:

Temperature:

Pulse:

Respiration:

Blood pressure (BP):

CVS, peripheral pulsations:

Respiratory system:

Gastrointestinal:

Musculoskeletal system:

Lymph nodes:

Breasts:

Pelvic examination:

Any other signs:

Summary:

Investigations

Name of the investigation	Patient value	Normal value	Remarks

Nursing Management

Nursing Assessment

Objective data:

Subjective data:

List of nursing diagnoses:

Nursing Care Plan

Assessment	Nursing diagnosis	Goal/objective	Intervention

Implementation	Rationale	Evaluation

Assessment	Nursing diagnosis	Goal/objective	Intervention

Implementation	Rationale	Evaluation

Medications

S. No.	Name of the drug	Dose and route	Mechanism of action	Adverse effects	Nurse's responsibility

Health education:

Conclusion:

Name and Signature of the Student   **Name and Signature of the Supervisor**

Proforma for Evaluating Care Plan in Psychiatric Nursing

Name of the student: Name of the patient:

Year: Hospital No.:

Register No.:   Age:

Area/ward: Sex:

Date of submission: Diagnosis:

S. No.	Criteria	Max. marks	Marks obtained
1.	Bio-data of the patient	½	
2.	Chief complaints	½	
3.	History of present illness	1	
4.	Past history	½	
5.	Personal history	1	
6.	Premorbid personality	½	
7.	Physical examination	1	
8.	Mental status examination	3	
9.	Nursing assessment data:		
	◆ Objective	½	
	◆ Subjective	½	
10.	Nursing diagnoses	2	
11.	Short-term goals and long-term goals	1	
12.	Plan of action with rationale	2	
13.	Implementation	2	
14.	Evaluation	1	
15.	Health education	2	
16.	Progress notes	1	
	Total	**20**	

Remarks:

Signature of the Student   **Signature of the Supervisor**

ASSIGNMENT - 14

Clinical/Case Presentation

Name of the student:

Year:

Group:

Size of group:

Venue:

Date and time:

Previous knowledge:

Methods of teaching:

AV aids:

General objectives:

Specific objectives:

Identification Data

Name:	Age:	Sex:

Name of the Father/Spouse:

Address:

Education:	Occupation:	Income:
Marital Status:	Religion:	

Informant:

Presenting Chief Complaint

History of Present Illness

Duration:

Mode of onset:

Course:

Intensity:

Precipitating factors:

Description of present illness:
While describing present illness consider chronological description of abnormal behavior, associated problems like suicide, homicide, disruptive behavior; thought content, speech, mood states, abnormal perception, biological functioning, social functioning, occupational functioning, changes in ADLs.

Past Psychiatric and Medical History

Family History

Name of the family member	Age	Education	Occupation	Health status	Relationship with the patient	Age at death and mode of death

Genogram (family of origin, three generations):

Personal History

A. Perinatal History

B. Childhood History

C. Educational History

D. Play History

E. Emotional Problems during Adolescence

F. Puberty

G. Obstetrical History

H. Occupational History

I. Sexual and Marital History

J. Premorbid Personality

Physical Examination

General examination:

Temperature:

Pulse:

Respiration:

Blood pressure (BP):

CVS, peripheral pulsations:

Respiratory system:

Gastrointestinal:

Musculoskeletal system:

Lymph nodes:

Breasts:

Pelvic examination:

Any other signs:

Summary:

Investigations

Name of the investigation	Patient value	Normal value	Remarks

Mental Status Examination

A. General Appearance and Behavior

Appearance:

Facial expression:

Level of grooming:

Level of cleanliness:

Level of consciousness:

Mode of entry:

Behavior:

Cooperativeness:

Eye-to-eye contact:

Psychomotor activity:

Rapport:

Gesturing:

Posturing:

Other movements:

Other catatonic phenomena:

Conversion and dissociative signs:

Hallucinatory behavior:

B. Speech

Initiation:

Reaction time:

Rate:

Productivity:

Volume:

Tone:

Relevance:

Stream (flow and rhythm of speech):

Coherence:

Others:

Sample of speech (in response to open-ended questions, verbatim in 2 or 3 sentences):

C. Mood and Affect

Subjective:

Objective:

Predominant mood state:

D. Thought

Stream (flow of thought):

Form (formal thought disorder):

Content:

E. Perception

Illusions:

Hallucinations (specify type and give example):

Somatic passivity:

Déjà vu/jamais vu:

Depersonalization/derealization:

F. Cognitive Function (Neuropsychiatric Assessment)

Consciousness:

Orientation:

- Time:

- Place:

- Person:

Attention:

- Digit forward:

- Digit backward:

Concentration:

Memory

- Immediate:

- Recent:

- Remote:

Intelligence

Abstraction

Judgment

G. Insight

Diagnostic Formulation

Book Picture of Disease Condition

Introduction

Definition

Incidence

Etiology

Book picture	Patient picture

Psychopathology

Clinical Manifestations

Book picture	Patient picture

Investigations

Book picture	Patient picture

Diagnosis

Treatment (psychopharmacological and psychosocial management)

Book picture	Patient picture

Nursing Management

Nursing Assessment

Objective data:

Subjective data:

List of nursing diagnoses:

Nursing Care Plan

Assessment	Nursing diagnosis	Goal/objective	Intervention

Implementation	Rationale	Evaluation

Assessment	Nursing diagnosis	Goal/objective	Intervention

Implementation	Rationale	Evaluation

Medications

S. No.	Name of the drug	Dose and route	Mechanism of action	Adverse effects	Nurse's responsibility

Health education:

Conclusion:

References:

Name and Signature of the Student   **Name and Signature of the Supervisor**

Proforma for Evaluating Clinical Presentation in Psychiatric Nursing

Name of the student: Name of the patient:

Year: Hospital No.:

Register No.: Age:

Area/ward: Sex:

Date of submission: Diagnosis:

S. No.	Criteria	Max. marks	Marks obtained
1.	History taking	2	
2.	Mental status examination	2	
3.	Description of diseased condition		
	• Definition	1	
	• Etiological factors	1	
	• Clinical manifestations (according to book and patient)	2	
4.	Diagnosis	1	
5.	Prognosis	1	
6.	Management		
	• Pharmacological therapy	1	
	• Psychological therapies	1	
	• Rehabilitation (according to book and patient)	1	
7.	Nursing management		
	• Nursing assessment	½	
	• Nursing diagnosis	1	
	• Planning	½	
	• Implementation	3	
	• Evaluation	½	
	• Health education	1	
8.	Bibliography	½	
	Total	**20**	

Remarks:

Signature of the Student **Signature of the Supervisor**

ASSIGNMENT - 15

Process Recording - I

I. Identification Data

Name: Age: Sex:

Religion: Marital Status: Educational status:

Occupation: Income per month: Languages known:

IP No.:   Ward: Diagnosis:

Address:

Date of admission: Date and time of process recording:

II. Brief Summary of the Patient Problem

III. Place of Interaction

IV. Description of the Environment

V. Reason for Selecting the Patient

VI. Objectives

1.

2.

3.

Nurse's response Verbal and non-verbal	Patient's response Verbal and non-verbal	Communication technique	Inference

Nurse's response Verbal and non-verbal	Patient's response Verbal and non-verbal	Communication technique	Inference

Conclusion—Fixing the time and place for the next interview:

List of inferences:

Any special difficulties faced during the inference:

Techniques used to overcome difficulties:

Name and Signature of the Student   **Name and Signature of the Supervisor**

Proforma for Evaluating Process Recording in Psychiatric Nursing

Name of the student:

Name of the patient:

Year:

Hospital No.:

Register No.:

Age:

Area/ward:

Sex:

Date of submission:

Diagnosis:

S. No.	Criteria	Max. marks	Marks obtained
1.	Identification data	½	
2.	Description of the environment	½	
3.	Objectives	1	
4.	Verbatim	1	
5.	Therapeutic techniques used	2	
	Total	**5**	

Remarks:

Signature of the Student

Signature of the Supervisor

ASSIGNMENT - 16

Process Recording - II

I. Identification Data

Name: Age: Sex:

Religion: Marital Status: Educational status:

Occupation: Income per month: Languages known:

IP No.:   Ward: Diagnosis:

Address:

Date of admission: Date and time of process recording:

II. Brief Summary of the Patient Problem

III. Place of Interaction

IV. Description of the Environment

V. Reason for Selecting the Patient

VI. Objectives

1.

2.

3.

Nurse's response Verbal and non-verbal	Patient's response Verbal and non-verbal	Communication technique	Inference

Nurse's response Verbal and non-verbal	Patient's response Verbal and non-verbal	Communication technique	Inference

Conclusion—Fixing the time and place for the next interview:

List of inferences:

Any special difficulties faced during the inference:

Techniques used to overcome difficulties:

Name and Signature of the Student   **Name and Signature of the Supervisor**

Proforma for Evaluating Process Recording in Psychiatric Nursing

Name of the student: Name of the patient:

Year: Hospital No.:

Register No.:   Age:

Area/ward: Sex:

Date of submission: Diagnosis:

S. No.	Criteria	Max. marks	Marks obtained
1.	Identification data	½	
2.	Description of the environment	½	
3.	Objectives	1	
4.	Verbatim	1	
5.	Therapeutic techniques used	2	
	Total	**5**	

Remarks:

Signature of the Student   **Signature of the Supervisor**

ASSIGNMENT - 17

Administration of Psychotropic Drugs - I

Demographic Data

Name of the patient: Age: Sex:

Religion: IP No.:   Marital status:

Education: Occupation:

Address:

Diagnosis:

Medical management:

Pharmacological name and trade name	Dose and route	Mechanism of action	Indications	Contraindications	Adverse effects	Nurse's responsibility

Pharmacological name and trade name	Dose and route	Mechanism of action	Indications	Contraindications	Adverse effects	Nurse's responsibility

References:

Signature of the Student

Signature of the Supervisor

ASSIGNMENT - 18

Administration of Psychotropic Drugs - II

Demographic Data

Name of the patient: Age: Sex:

Religion: IP No.:   Marital status:

Education: Occupation:

Address:

Diagnosis:

Medical management:

Pharmacological name and trade name	Dose and route	Mechanism of action	Indications	Contraindications	Adverse effects	Nurse's responsibility

Pharmacological name and trade name	Dose and route	Mechanism of action	Indications	Contraindications	Adverse effects	Nurse's responsibility

References:

Signature of the Student

Signature of the Supervisor

ASSIGNMENT - 19

Administration of Psychotropic Drugs - III

Demographic Data

Name of the patient: Age: Sex:

Religion: IP No.:   Marital status:

Education: Occupation:

Address:

Diagnosis:

Medical management:

Pharmacological name and trade name	Dose and route	Mechanism of action	Indications	Contraindications	Adverse effects	Nurse's responsibility

Pharmacological name and trade name	Dose and route	Mechanism of action	Indications	Contraindications	Adverse effects	Nurse's responsibility

References:

Signature of the Student   Signature of the Supervisor

ASSIGNMENT - 20

Assist the Patient for Electroconvulsive Therapy

I. Identification Data

Name of the patient: Age: Sex:

Religion: IP No.:   Marital status:

Education: Occupation:

Address:

Informant:

II. Presenting Chief Complaints

III. Brief Description of the Patient Illness

IV. Mental Status Examination

General appearance and behavior:

Speech:

Mood:

Thought:

Perception:

Cognitive function:

Insight:

Judgment:

Diagnostic formulation:

V. Physical Examination

VI. Assessment of Patient's and Family's Knowledge of Indications, Side Effects, Therapeutic Effects and Risks Associated with ECT

VII. Pre ECT Care Checklist

S. No.	Particulars	Yes/No
1.	Informed consent	
2.	Assess vital signs	
3.	Nil by mouth (6–8 hours)	
4.	Withhold night dose of drugs	
5.	Withhold oral medications in the morning	
6.	Head shampooing	
7.	Remove jewels, prosthesis, dentures, contact lens, etc.	
8.	Remove tight clothing	
9.	Empty bladder and bowel just before ECT	
10.	Pre ECT medications	

VIII. Intra-procedure Care Checklist

S. No.	Particulars	Yes/No
1.	Place the patient comfortably on the ECT table	
2.	Stay with the patient	
3.	Insert mouth gag	
4.	Apply gel and electrodes	
5.	Monitor voltage intensity and duration of electrical activity	
6.	Monitor seizure activity	
7.	Monitor vital signs	

IX. Post-procedure Care Checklist

S. No.	Particulars	Yes/No
1.	Place patient in sideline position	
2.	Monitor vital signs	
3.	Oxygen administration	
4.	Assess for post ictal confusion	
5.	Use of side rails to prevent falls	
6.	Re-orient the patient after recovery	
7.	Recording the case	

Summary

List the equipment available in ECT room

List the medications available in ECT room

Describe the staffing pattern and duty timings of the staff

Draw and describe the physical layout of the ECT room

Name and Signature of the Student   **Name and Signature of the Supervisor**

ASSIGNMENT - 21

Assist the Patient for Individual Psychotherapy

I. Demographic Data

Name of the patient: Age: Sex:

Religion: IP No.:   Marital status:

Education: Occupation:

Address:

Informant:

II. Brief Description of the Patient Illness

III. Brief Description of Mental Status Examination

IV. Treatment History

V. Indications for Psychotherapy

VI. Problems Identified for Work Up

VII. Brief Description of Psychotherapy given to the Patient

Session No.:

Place:

Time:

Psychotherapy approach:

Techniques used by the therapist:

Plan for next session:

Home works, if any (given to the patient):

Outcome of the session:

Summary

Name and Signature of the Student   **Name and Signature of the Supervisor**

ASSIGNMENT - 22

Assist the Patient for Family Psychotherapy

I. Demographic Data

Name of the patient: Age: Sex:

Religion: IP No.:   Marital status:

Education: Occupation:

Address:

Informant:

II. Brief Description of the Patient Illness

III. Brief Description of Mental Status Examination

IV. Treatment History

V. Indications for Family Psychotherapy

VI. Brief Description of Family Psychotherapy given to the Patient

Session No.:

Place:

Time:

List the family members who participated in therapy:

Communication pattern among family members:

Family therapy approach:

Techniques used by the therapist:

Plan for next session:

Home works, if any (given to the patient):

Outcome of the session:

Summary

Name and Signature of the Student   **Name and Signature of the Supervisor**

ASSIGNMENT - 23

Assist the Patient for Group Psychotherapy

I. Demographic Data

Name of the patient: Age: Sex:

Religion: IP No.:   Marital status:

Education: Occupation:

Address:

Informant:

II. Brief Description of the Patient Illness

III. Brief Description of Mental Status Examination

IV. Treatment History

V. Indications for Group Psychotherapy

VI. Group Size

VII. Topics Addressed in Group Therapy

VIII. Techniques Used in Group Therapy

IX. Problems Encountered in the Group Therapy

X. Summary of Group Therapy

Signature of the Student   **Signature of the Supervisor**

ASSIGNMENT - 24

Assist the Patient for Occupational Psychotherapy

I. Demographic Data

Name of the patient:	Age:	Sex:
Religion:	IP No.:	Marital status:
Education:	Occupation:	
Address:		
Informant:		

II. Brief Description of the Patient Illness

III. Brief Description of Mental Status Examination

IV. Treatment History

V. Objective for Occupational Therapy

VI. Evaluation of the Patient

Current level of functioning:

Social functioning:

Behavioral problems:

VII. Description of Occupational Therapy (Activities) Planned or Provided for Patient

Description of activities	Therapeutic value

Summary (Focus on difficulties faced by the patient during therapy, outcome of the session and plan for the next session)

Signature of the Student   **Signature of the Supervisor**

ASSIGNMENT - 25

Assist the Patient for Behavioral Psychotherapy

I. Demographic Data

Name of the patient: Age: Sex:

Religion: IP No.:   Marital status:

Education: Occupation:

Address:

Informant:

II. Brief Description of the Patient Illness

III. Brief Description of Mental Status Examination

IV. Treatment History

V. Indications for Behavioral Therapy

VI. Techniques Used by the Therapist

VII. Summary of Behavior Therapy

Signature of the Student   **Signature of the Supervisor**

ASSIGNMENT - 26

Assist the Patient for Recreational Therapy

I. Demographic Data

Name of the patient: Age: Sex:

Religion: IP No.:   Marital status:

Education: Occupation:

Address:

Informant:

II. Brief Description of the Patient Illness

III. Brief Description of Mental Status Examination

IV. Treatment History

V. Indications for Recreational Therapy

VI. Advantages of Therapy for the Patient

VII. Summary of Recreational Therapy Provided for Patient in the Ward

Signature of the Student   **Signature of the Supervisor**

ASSIGNMENT - 27

Assist the Patient for Play Therapy

I. Demographic Data

Name of the patient: Age: Sex:

Religion: IP No.:   Marital status:

Education: Occupation:

Address:

Informant:

II. Brief Description of the Patient Illness

III. Brief Description of Mental Status Examination

IV. Treatment History

V. Indications for Play Therapy

VI. Advantages of Therapy for the Patient

VII. Summary of Play Therapy Provided for Patient in the Ward

Signature of the Student   **Signature of the Supervisor**

ASSIGNMENT - 28

Preparation of Patients for Activities of Daily Living - I

Name of the patient: Age: Sex:

Religion: IP No.:   Marital status:

Education: Occupation:

Address:

Diagnosis:

Assess for Self-care Ability

- **Patient is concerned about keeping clean:** Totally unconcerned/occasionally concerned/always concerned
- **Patient is concerned about eating right food:** Totally unconcerned/occasionally concerned/always concerned
- **Patient is concerned with daily activities:** Totally unconcerned/occasionally concerned/always concerned

List Nursing Diagnosis

List Nursing Interventions Related to Activities of Daily Living

Evaluation:

Signature of the Student   **Signature of the Supervisor**

ASSIGNMENT - 29

Preparation of Patients for Activities of Daily Living - II

Name of the patient: Age: Sex:

Religion: IP No.:   Marital status:

Education: Occupation:

Address:

Diagnosis:

Assess for Self-care Ability

- **Patient is concerned about keeping clean:** Totally unconcerned/occasionally concerned/always concerned
- **Patient is concerned about eating right food:** Totally unconcerned/occasionally concerned/always concerned
- **Patient is concerned with daily activities:** Totally unconcerned/occasionally concerned/always concerned

List Nursing Diagnosis

List Nursing Interventions Related to Activities of Daily Living

Evaluation:

Signature of the Student   **Signature of the Supervisor**

ASSIGNMENT - 30

Preparation of Patients for Activities of Daily Living - III

Name of the patient: Age: Sex:

Religion: IP No.:   Marital status:

Education: Occupation:

Address:

Diagnosis:

Assess for Self-care Ability

- **Patient is concerned about keeping clean:** Totally unconcerned/occasionally concerned/always concerned
- **Patient is concerned about eating right food:** Totally unconcerned/occasionally concerned/always concerned
- **Patient is concerned with daily activities:** Totally unconcerned/occasionally concerned/always concerned

List Nursing Diagnosis

List Nursing Interventions Related to Activities of Daily Living

Evaluation:

Signature of the Student   **Signature of the Supervisor**

ASSIGNMENT - 31

Admission Procedure

Date:

Name:

Education:

Age:

Occupation and income:

Sex:

Marital status:

Date of admission:

Hospital No.:

Diagnosis:

Address:

Nursing interventions given to patient
Type of admission
Mention whether consent was given by patient/family member/any other
Brief description of patient condition
Brief description on preparation of patient unit

Describe the preparation of patient record with all the information like unit, bed number, weight, vital signs, MSE and general condition, etc., and write the admission note with details such as time of patient arrival to ward, mode of arrival, patient's complaints, and any other significant information

Describe the orientation given to the patient regarding physical set up of the ward, hospital policies regarding meal time, ward activities, visiting hours, gate pass, attendant staying with the patient and restrictions in the ward

List the investigations advised such as urine, blood or any other

List the medications ordered by the psychiatrist with details (dose, route and frequency)

Name and Signature of the Student **Name and Signature of the Supervisor**

ASSIGNMENT - 32

Discharge Procedure

Name:

Age:

Sex:

Date of admission:

Diagnosis:

Address:

Date:

Education:

Occupation and income:

Marital status:

Hospital No.:

Nursing interventions given to patient
Type of discharge
Check for physician's discharge order
Assess and describe the patient's health care needs at the time of discharge
Write a note on discharge summary

List the medications prescribed to the patient as ordered by the psychiatrist

Write a note on follow-up visits

Brief description of health education provided to the patient

Summary of nurse's notes

Name and Signature of the Student   **Name and Signature of the Supervisor**

ASSIGNMENT - 33

Health Education

Name of the topic:

Group and number:

Place:

Date and time:

Duration of health education:

Name of the student:

Name of the supervisor:

Method of teaching:

AV aids:

General objectives:

Specific objectives:

Specific objective	Content	AV aids	Evaluation

Specific objective	Content	AV aids	Evaluation

Specific objective	Content	AV aids	Evaluation

Specific objective	Content	AV aids	Evaluation

References:

Name and Signature of the Student

Name and Signature of the Supervisor

ASSIGNMENT - 34

Psychotropic Drug Book

Pharmacological name and trade name	Dose and route	Mechanism of action	Indications	Contra-indications	Adverse effects	Nurse's responsibility

Pharmacological name and trade name	Dose and route	Mechanism of action	Indications	Contra-indications	Adverse effects	Nurse's responsibility

Pharmacological name and trade name	Dose and route	Mechanism of action	Indications	Contra-indications	Adverse effects	Nurse's responsibility

Pharmacological name and trade name	Dose and route	Mechanism of action	Indications	Contra-indications	Adverse effects	Nurse's responsibility

Pharmacological name and trade name	Dose and route	Mechanism of action	Indications	Contra-indications	Adverse effects	Nurse's responsibility

Pharmacological name and trade name	Dose and route	Mechanism of action	Indications	Contra-indications	Adverse effects	Nurse's responsibility

Pharmacological name and trade name	Dose and route	Mechanism of action	Indications	Contra-indications	Adverse effects	Nurse's responsibility

Pharmacological name and trade name	Dose and route	Mechanism of action	Indications	Contra-indications	Adverse effects	Nurse's responsibility

Pharmacological name and trade name	Dose and route	Mechanism of action	Indications	Contra-indications	Adverse effects	Nurse's responsibility

Pharmacological name and trade name	Dose and route	Mechanism of action	Indications	Contra-indications	Adverse effects	Nurse's responsibility

Pharmacological name and trade name	Dose and route	Mechanism of action	Indications	Contra-indications	Adverse effects	Nurse's responsibility

Pharmacological name and trade name	Dose and route	Mechanism of action	Indications	Contra-indications	Adverse effects	Nurse's responsibility

Pharmacological name and trade name	Dose and route	Mechanism of action	Indications	Contra-indications	Adverse effects	Nurse's responsibility

Pharmacological name and trade name	Dose and route	Mechanism of action	Indications	Contra-indications	Adverse effects	Nurse's responsibility

Pharmacological name and trade name	Dose and route	Mechanism of action	Indications	Contra-indications	Adverse effects	Nurse's responsibility

Pharmacological name and trade name	Dose and route	Mechanism of action	Indications	Contra-indications	Adverse effects	Nurse's responsibility

Pharmacological name and trade name	Dose and route	Mechanism of action	Indications	Contra-indications	Adverse effects	Nurse's responsibility

Pharmacological name and trade name	Dose and route	Mechanism of action	Indications	Contra-indications	Adverse effects	Nurse's responsibility

Pharmacological name and trade name	Dose and route	Mechanism of action	Indications	Contra-indications	Adverse effects	Nurse's responsibility

Pharmacological name and trade name	Dose and route	Mechanism of action	Indications	Contra-indications	Adverse effects	Nurse's responsibility

ASSIGNMENT - 35

Community Case Work

1. Geographic Assessment

Name of the place/area:

Rural/urban:

Name of the PHC/sub-center:

2. Family Identification Information

Name of the head of the family:

Nature of the family : nuclear/joint:

Religion:

Caste:

Address:

3. Family Characteristics and Health Status of the Family Members

Sl. No.	Name of the family member	Age	Sex	Relationship with the head of the family	Education and occupation	Health status
1.						
2.						
3.						
4.						
5.						
6.						

4. Housing Condition

- Type of house : Pucca/kutcha/mixed
- Number of rooms :
- Ventilation : Adequate/inadequate
- Lighting : Electricity/lamp
- Water supply : Tap/hand/bore-well/well/any other specify
- Kitchen : Separate/corner of the room
- Smoke outlet : Yes/no
- Bathroom : Yes/no
- Latrine : Own/public/open air defecation
- Drainage : Open/closed
- Refuse disposal : Dumping/burning/any other specify
- Cattle shed : Yes/no
- If yes, distance from home :

Utilization of health services: PHC/private services/Govt. hospital/nursing home/any other specify

5. Socioeconomic Status

- House : Own/rented
- Land : Yes/no
- Main occupation :
- Income of the family per month :
- Facilities at home : TV/radio/VCR/refrigerator/phone/computer/any other specify

6. Transport and Communication

- Type of road : Tar road/mud road
- Transport facilities : Bus/auto/any other specify
- Communication facilities : Radio/newspaper/magazine/TV/computer/phone any other specify

7. Nutritional Pattern

- Food habits : Vegetarian/non-vegetarian
- Specify any nutritional deficiencies :
- Summary of nutritional intake (quantity and quality) of family members:

8. Assessment of Support System

- Relationship with neighbors   : Good/moderate/minimum/absent
- Relationship with relatives   : Good/moderate/minimum/absent

9. Assessment of Risk Factors for Mental Health

S. No.	Name of the family member	Present health status	Any chronic diseases	Specify any stressors
1.				
2.				
3.				
4.				
5.				
6.				

- Family history of mental illness
- Use of leisure time
- Recreational activities/relaxation activities
- Describe cultural practices related to health
- Describe religious practices/festivals
- Interpersonal relationship among family members: Adequate/inadequate
- Any addictions: Chewing *paan*/smoking/alcoholism/drug addiction/snuff/any other specify
- Vital occurrences during last one year: Marriage/birth/death (cause)/new job/education related changes
- History of past significant illnesses and accidents
- Physical handicap: Present/absent, if present, specify
- Mental retardation: Present/absent, if present, specify degree of retardation
- History of epilepsy/suicide

Knowledge of the family about mental health and illness: Good/moderate/poor, specify briefly:

Attitude of the family about mental health and mental illness: Positive/negative, specify briefly:

Nursing Care Plan

Health Problems Perceived by the Family

1.

2.

3.

4.

5.

6.

Health Problems Perceived by the Student

1.

2.

3.

4.

5.

6.

List down the Priority Mental Health Needs of the Family

1.

2.

3.

4.

5.

6.

Nursing Actions

1.

2.

3.

4.

5.

6.

Evaluation

Summary of Family Visit

Name and Signature of the Student

Name and Signature of the Supervisor

ASSIGNMENT - 36

Observational Report on Field Visits

Name of the community area:

Date of visit:

List the objectives of visit:

1.

2.

3.

4.

List various services provided in the community:

1.

2.

3.

4.

List the various organizations visited with date and address:

1.

2.

3.

4.

List the common psychiatric conditions found in the community:

Describe psychological first aid management provided to each condition:

Give a brief account of learning experience achieved from this field visit:

Name and Signature of the Student   **Name and Signature of the Supervisor**

Observational Report on Community Mental Health Center

Name of the community mental health center:

Date of visit:

Describe location of center:

When, where and how did this institution originate?

List the objectives of community mental health center:

1.

2.

3.

4.

5.

List various services provided by the center:

1.

2.

3.

4.

5.

Mention the various departments existing in the center:

1.

2.

3.

4.

5.

Draw the organizational structure of the center:

What are the staffing pattern and duty timings for the nurses?

Briefly describe the physical set-up:

Give a brief account of learning experience achieved from this visit

Name and Signature of the Student   **Name and Signature of the Supervisor**

ASSIGNMENT - 37

Observational Report on De-addiction Center

Name of the de-addiction center:

Date of visit:

When, where and how did this institution originate?

Describe philosophy of the organization

List the objectives:

1.

2.

3.

4.

5.

List various services provided by the organization

1.

2.

3.

4.

5.

Mention the various departments existing in the organization

1.

2.

3.

4.

5.

Draw the organizational structure of the center

Describe staffing pattern and duty timings of the staff:

Briefly describe the physical set-up:

Describe admission procedure:

Describe discharge procedure:

Explain activity schedule of inmates in the de-addiction center:

Describe recreational activities provided in the de-addiction center:

Give a brief account of learning experience achieved from this visit:

Name and Signature of the Student   **Name and Signature of the Supervisor**